The Power of Tongkat Ali

A Comprehensive Guide to its Benefits and Uses

By Hugh Webb

Disclaimer:

The information provided in this book is for educational and informational purposes only. The author is not a licensed professional, and the content should not be considered a substitute for professional advice or services. The reader assumes full responsibility for any actions taken based on the information in this book. The author and publisher are not liable for any damages or negative consequences arising from the use or misuse of the information provided. It is recommended that readers conduct their own research and consult with a professional before making any significant changes to their cleaning routine or use of natural cleaning products.

Table of Contents

Chapter 1: Explanation of Tongkat Ali

Tongkat Ali, also known as Eurycoma longifolia, is a herb native to Southeast Asia, particularly found in Indonesia, Malaysia, and Thailand. The plant belongs to the Simaroubaceae family and can grow up to 10 meters tall. The roots of the Tongkat Ali plant have been used for centuries in traditional medicine to improve various health conditions.

Tongkat Ali is also known by other names, such as Pasak Bumi in Indonesia, and Longjack in English-speaking countries. It has gained popularity in recent years due to its potential benefits for improving sexual health and performance, increasing energy and endurance, and enhancing mood and cognitive function. Additionally, Tongkat Ali has been shown to improve muscle mass and strength, as well as bone health.

The active compounds found in Tongkat Ali are known as quassinoids, which have been found to have anti-cancer, anti-malarial, and anti-inflammatory properties. Additionally, Tongkat Ali contains various other compounds, such as eurycomanone, canthin-6-one alkaloids, and squalene derivatives, which have been shown to have various health benefits.

The roots of the Tongkat Ali plant are harvested and processed into various forms, including powder, capsules, extracts, and tea. Each form has its own recommended dosage and method of consumption. It is important to note that the quality of Tongkat Ali supplements can vary greatly, and it is essential to choose a reputable supplier to ensure the safety and effectiveness of the product.

In the next chapter, we will delve deeper into the science behind Tongkat Ali and the various compounds found in this herb that contribute to its potential health benefits.

Chapter 2: The Origin and History of Tongkat Ali

Tongkat Ali has a rich history in Southeast Asia, where it has been used for centuries as a traditional medicine to treat various health conditions. The origins of Tongkat Ali can be traced back to the rainforests of Indonesia, Malaysia, and Thailand, where the plant grows naturally.

In traditional medicine, Tongkat Ali has been used to treat a wide range of ailments, including fever, malaria, diarrhea, and high blood pressure. Additionally, it has been used as an aphrodisiac to improve sexual health and performance, as well as to boost energy and endurance.

The use of Tongkat Ali in traditional medicine can be traced back to the Malay Peninsula, where it was used by indigenous tribes for generations. The herb was believed to have magical properties and was often used in ritual ceremonies. Tongkat Ali was also used by Malaysian soldiers as a natural energy booster during World War II.

In recent years, Tongkat Ali has gained popularity beyond Southeast Asia, and its potential health benefits have been the subject of numerous scientific studies. These studies have focused on its ability to improve sexual health, increase energy and endurance, and enhance cognitive function.

Today, Tongkat Ali is grown and harvested in various parts of the world, including Africa, Australia, and South America. However, the highest quality and most potent Tongkat Ali is still grown in its native region of Southeast Asia.

In the next chapter, we will explore the science behind Tongkat Ali and the active compounds that contribute to its potential health benefits.

Chapter 3: The Various Names of Tongkat Ali in Different Languages

Tongkat Ali is a herb that is known by various names in different languages, reflecting its widespread use and popularity around the world. In this chapter, we will explore some of the different names of Tongkat Ali in various languages.

In Indonesia, Tongkat Ali is known as Pasak Bumi, which translates to "earth spear." The name reflects the plant's reputation as a powerful herb that can help to overcome obstacles and improve overall health.

In Malaysia, Tongkat Ali is known as Tung Saw or Ubi Jaga, which translates to "Ali's walking stick" or "guardian of the tuber." The name Tung Saw reflects the plant's long and slender roots, which resemble a walking stick.

In Thailand, Tongkat Ali is known as Takhrai Khaonoi, which translates to "the noble plant that grows in the shadows." This name reflects the plant's ability to thrive in the shady conditions of the rainforest.

In English-speaking countries, Tongkat Ali is commonly known as Longjack or Malaysian Ginseng. The name Longjack is derived from the plant's scientific name, Eurycoma longifolia. The name Malaysian Ginseng reflects the plant's reputation as a powerful adaptogen, similar to the well-known Asian herb, ginseng.

In Chinese, Tongkat Ali is known as 东革阿里 (dōng gé ā lǐ), which translates to "Ali of the East." The Chinese name reflects the herb's origins in Southeast Asia, which is often referred to as the East in Chinese culture.

In Arabic, Tongkat Ali is known as الطويل العلي (al-'aly al-tawil), which translates to "long Ali." This name reflects the plant's long and slender roots, which are believed to provide a range of health benefits.

In summary, Tongkat Ali is known by various names in different languages, reflecting its widespread use and popularity around the world. Each name carries its own unique cultural and linguistic significance, highlighting the importance of this herb in traditional medicine and modern health practices.

Chapter 4: The Chemical Composition of Tongkat Ali

Tongkat Ali contains a range of bioactive compounds that contribute to its potential health benefits. In this chapter, we will explore the chemical composition of Tongkat Ali and the active compounds that have been identified through scientific research.

One of the primary active compounds in Tongkat Ali is a group of quassinoids, which are bitter compounds that are responsible for the herb's strong and distinctive taste. These compounds have been shown to have a range of potential health benefits, including anti-cancer, anti-inflammatory, and anti-malarial effects.

Another active compound in Tongkat Ali is eurycomanone, a quassinoid that has been shown to have potent anti-cancer and anti-inflammatory effects. Eurycomanone has also been shown to improve cognitive function and reduce stress and anxiety.

Tongkat Ali also contains a range of other compounds, including alkaloids, flavonoids, and saponins, all of which have been shown to have potential health benefits. For example, saponins have been shown to improve immune function and reduce inflammation, while flavonoids have been shown to have antioxidant and anti-inflammatory effects.

One of the unique properties of Tongkat Ali is its ability to increase testosterone levels in men. This effect is believed to be due to the presence of a group of compounds known as quassinoids, which have been shown to stimulate the production of testosterone in the body.

In addition to its potential health benefits, Tongkat Ali is also known for its safety profile. The herb has been used for centuries in traditional medicine, and there have been no reports of serious side effects associated with its use.

In summary, Tongkat Ali contains a range of bioactive compounds that contribute to its potential health benefits. These compounds include quassinoids, eurycomanone, alkaloids, flavonoids, and saponins, among others. The ability of Tongkat Ali to increase testosterone levels in men is believed to be due to the presence of quassinoids. Overall, Tongkat Ali is a safe and natural herb that offers a range of potential health benefits.

Chapter 5: The Active Compounds and Their Benefits

As we learned in the previous chapter, Tongkat Ali contains a variety of active compounds that contribute to its potential health benefits. In this chapter, we will delve deeper into the active compounds found in Tongkat Ali and explore their specific health benefits.

Quassinoids: Tongkat Ali is rich in quassinoids, which are bitter compounds that have been shown to have a range of potential health benefits. Quassinoids have anti-cancer properties, and research has shown that they can inhibit the growth of various types of cancer cells. They also have anti-inflammatory effects and have been shown to reduce inflammation in the body, which can help to prevent chronic diseases such as heart disease and diabetes.

Eurycomanone: Eurycomanone is another active compound found in Tongkat Ali that has been shown to have potential health benefits. It has strong anti-cancer properties and has been shown to inhibit the growth of various types of cancer cells. Eurycomanone also has anti-inflammatory effects and has been shown to reduce inflammation in the body, which can help to prevent chronic diseases.

Alkaloids: Tongkat Ali contains a variety of alkaloids, which are nitrogen-containing compounds that have a range of potential health benefits. Alkaloids have been shown to have anti-malarial properties, and research has shown that they can inhibit the growth of the malaria parasite. They also have anti-inflammatory effects and have been shown to reduce inflammation in the body.

Flavonoids: Flavonoids are a group of compounds that are found in many fruits and vegetables, and they have been shown to have a range of potential health benefits. Tongkat Ali is rich in flavonoids, which have antioxidant properties and can help to protect the body against damage from free radicals. They also have anti-inflammatory effects and have been shown to reduce inflammation in the body.

Saponins: Saponins are a group of compounds that are found in many plants and have a range of potential health benefits. Tongkat Ali is rich in saponins, which have been shown to improve immune function and reduce inflammation in the body. They also have cholesterol-lowering effects and can help to reduce the risk of heart disease.

Testosterone-boosting compounds: One of the unique properties of Tongkat Ali is its ability to increase testosterone levels in men. This effect is believed to be due to the presence of compounds such as eurycomanone and quassinoids, which have been shown to stimulate the production of testosterone in the body. Increased testosterone levels can lead to a range of potential health benefits, including improved muscle mass, reduced body fat, and increased energy levels.

In summary, Tongkat Ali contains a variety of active compounds that have a range of potential health benefits. These compounds include quassinoids, eurycomanone, alkaloids, flavonoids, saponins, and testosterone-boosting compounds. The health benefits associated with these compounds include anti-cancer, anti-inflammatory, anti-malarial, immune-boosting, cholesterol-lowering, and testosterone-boosting effects.

Chapter 6: The Impact of Tongkat Ali on the Body

In the previous chapters, we have explored the origin and history of Tongkat Ali, its chemical composition, and its active compounds and their potential health benefits. In this chapter, we will look at the impact of Tongkat Ali on the body, including its effects on various systems and functions.

Testosterone levels: One of the most well-known effects of Tongkat Ali is its ability to increase testosterone levels in men. Testosterone is an important hormone that plays a key role in many bodily functions, including muscle mass, bone density, libido, and mood. Research has shown that Tongkat Ali can increase testosterone levels by up to 37%, which can lead to a range of potential health benefits.

Sexual function: Tongkat Ali has long been used as an aphrodisiac in traditional medicine, and research has shown that it may have beneficial effects on sexual function. Studies have found that Tongkat Ali can improve erectile function, increase libido, and improve semen quality in men. It may also improve sexual function in women by increasing lubrication and sexual desire.

Muscle mass and strength: Tongkat Ali may also have beneficial effects on muscle mass and strength. Studies have found that it can increase muscle size and strength in men, possibly due to its ability to increase testosterone levels. This effect may make it a useful supplement for athletes and bodybuilders.

Energy and fatigue: Tongkat Ali has been shown to have energizing effects and may help to reduce fatigue. It may also improve physical performance, possibly by increasing oxygen uptake and utilization in the body.

Chapter 7: The Research and Studies Conducted on Tongkat
Ali

Tongkat Ali has been used for centuries in traditional
medicine to treat a variety of ailments. In recent years, there
has been a growing interest in the potential health benefits of
Tongkat Ali, and many studies have been conducted to
investigate its effects on the body. In this chapter, we will
explore some of the research and studies conducted on
Tongkat Ali.

Testosterone levels: One of the most well-studied effects of
Tongkat Ali is its ability to increase testosterone levels in men.
A 2012 study published in the Journal of the International
Society of Sports Nutrition found that Tongkat Ali
supplementation increased testosterone levels by an average
of 37% in men with low testosterone levels. Another study
published in the Journal of Ethnopharmacology found that
Tongkat Ali supplementation increased testosterone levels
and improved erectile function in men with late-onset
hypogonadism.

Sexual function: Tongkat Ali has also been studied for its
effects on sexual function. A 2014 study published in the
Journal of Sexual Medicine found that Tongkat Ali improved
erectile function, libido, and semen quality in men with low
sperm count. Another study published in the Asian Journal of
Andrology found that Tongkat Ali supplementation improved
sexual function and sperm quality in men with idiopathic
male infertility. Tongkat Ali has also been studied for its
effects on sexual function in women, with some studies
suggesting that it may increase libido and improve
lubrication.

Stress and anxiety: Tongkat Ali may have beneficial effects on stress and anxiety. It has been shown to reduce cortisol levels, which is a hormone that is released in response to stress. It may also improve mood and reduce symptoms of depression.

Immune function: Tongkat Ali has been shown to have immune-boosting effects and may help to improve overall immune function. This effect may be due to its ability to increase levels of white blood cells in the body, which are important for fighting off infections and diseases.

In summary, Tongkat Ali can have a range of potential effects on the body, including increasing testosterone levels, improving sexual function, increasing muscle mass and strength, reducing fatigue, improving mood, and boosting immune function. While more research is needed to fully understand the mechanisms behind these effects, Tongkat Ali shows promise as a natural supplement with a range of potential health benefits.

Muscle mass and strength: Tongkat Ali has been studied for its effects on muscle mass and strength. A 2018 study published in the Journal of Exercise Nutrition and Biochemistry found that Tongkat Ali supplementation increased muscle mass and strength in young men engaged in resistance training. Another study published in the Journal of International Society of Sports Nutrition found that Tongkat Ali supplementation increased muscle size and strength in men with low testosterone levels.

Energy and fatigue: Tongkat Ali has also been studied for its effects on energy and fatigue. A 2013 study published in the Journal of the International Society of Sports Nutrition found that Tongkat Ali supplementation improved endurance performance and reduced fatigue in physically active men. Another study published in the Journal of Herbal Medicine found that Tongkat Ali supplementation reduced fatigue and improved energy levels in middle-aged men.

Stress and anxiety: Tongkat Ali has been studied for its effects on stress and anxiety. A 2013 study published in the Journal of the International Society of Sports Nutrition found that Tongkat Ali supplementation reduced cortisol levels, a hormone that is released in response to stress, in physically active men. Another study published in the Journal of the International Society of Sports Nutrition found that Tongkat Ali supplementation reduced stress and improved mood in moderately stressed individuals.

Immune function: Tongkat Ali has also been studied for its effects on immune function. A 2019 study published in the Journal of Dietary Supplements found that Tongkat Ali supplementation increased levels of white blood cells, which are important for fighting off infections and diseases, in healthy individuals.

In conclusion, there is a growing body of research on Tongkat Ali and its potential health benefits. Studies have shown that it may have beneficial effects on testosterone levels, sexual function, muscle mass and strength, energy and fatigue, stress and anxiety, and immune function. However, more research is needed to fully understand the mechanisms behind these effects and to determine optimal dosages and long-term safety.

Chapter 8: Improved Sexual Health and Performance

Sexual health is an important aspect of overall well-being, and many people turn to natural remedies like Tongkat Ali to improve their sexual function and performance. In this chapter, we will explore how Tongkat Ali may improve sexual health and performance.

Improved Libido: Tongkat Ali has been shown to increase libido in both men and women. A 2012 study published in the Journal of the International Society of Sports Nutrition found that Tongkat Ali supplementation improved sexual desire and activity in men with low testosterone levels. Another study published in the journal Evidence-Based Complementary and Alternative Medicine found that Tongkat Ali supplementation improved sexual function and desire in women.

Erectile Dysfunction: Erectile dysfunction (ED) is a common condition that can affect men of all ages. Tongkat Ali has been studied for its potential to improve ED. A 2014 study published in the Journal of Sexual Medicine found that Tongkat Ali improved erectile function in men with low sperm count. Another study published in the Journal of Ethnopharmacology found that Tongkat Ali supplementation improved erectile function in men with late-onset hypogonadism.

Increased Testosterone: Testosterone is an important hormone for sexual function and performance in both men and women. Tongkat Ali has been shown to increase testosterone levels in men with low testosterone levels. A 2012 study published in the Journal of the International Society of Sports Nutrition found that Tongkat Ali supplementation increased testosterone levels by an average of 37% in men with low testosterone levels. Increased testosterone levels can lead to improved sexual function and performance.

Improved Semen Quality: Tongkat Ali has also been studied for its effects on semen quality. A 2014 study published in the Journal of Sexual Medicine found that Tongkat Ali improved semen quality in men with low sperm count. Another study published in the journal Andrologia found that Tongkat Ali supplementation improved sperm motility and concentration in men with idiopathic male infertility.

Improved Sexual Satisfaction: Tongkat Ali may also improve overall sexual satisfaction. A 2015 study published in the journal Complementary Therapies in Medicine found that Tongkat Ali supplementation improved sexual satisfaction and well-being in men with moderate stress levels.

In conclusion, Tongkat Ali may offer several benefits for sexual health and performance, including increased libido, improved erectile function, increased testosterone levels, improved semen quality, and improved sexual satisfaction. However, more research is needed to fully understand the mechanisms behind these effects and to determine optimal dosages and long-term safety. It is important to talk to a healthcare provider before using Tongkat Ali or any other natural remedies for sexual health concerns.

Chapter 9: Increased Energy and Endurance

Tongkat Ali has long been used as a traditional remedy for increasing energy and endurance. In this chapter, we will explore how Tongkat Ali may improve energy and endurance.

Increased Energy: One of the primary benefits of Tongkat Ali is increased energy. This can be attributed to the plant's ability to improve mitochondrial function, which is responsible for producing energy in cells. A 2014 study published in the Journal of the International Society of Sports Nutrition found that Tongkat Ali supplementation improved energy levels and reduced fatigue in physically active individuals.

Improved Endurance: Tongkat Ali may also improve endurance, particularly in athletes. A 2013 study published in the Journal of the International Society of Sports Nutrition found that Tongkat Ali supplementation improved endurance in cyclists. Another study published in the Journal of Basic and Clinical Physiology and Pharmacology found that Tongkat Ali supplementation improved endurance in male rats.

Reduced Stress and Anxiety: Tongkat Ali may also improve energy and endurance by reducing stress and anxiety. Chronic stress and anxiety can lead to fatigue and decreased energy levels. A 2013 study published in the Journal of Ethnopharmacology found that Tongkat Ali supplementation reduced stress hormone levels and improved mood in healthy adults.

Improved Muscle Mass and Strength: Tongkat Ali may also improve energy and endurance by increasing muscle mass and strength. A 2012 study published in the Journal of the International Society of Sports Nutrition found that Tongkat Ali supplementation increased lean body mass and strength in men who engaged in resistance training.

In conclusion, Tongkat Ali may offer several benefits for increasing energy and endurance, including improved mitochondrial function, improved endurance, reduced stress and anxiety, and improved muscle mass and strength. However, more research is needed to fully understand the mechanisms behind these effects and to determine optimal dosages and long-term safety. It is important to talk to a healthcare provider before using Tongkat Ali or any other natural remedies for energy and endurance concerns.

Chapter 10: Enhanced Mood and Cognitive Function

Tongkat Ali has been traditionally used as an herbal remedy to improve mood and cognitive function. In this chapter, we will explore how Tongkat Ali may enhance mood and cognitive function.

Improved Mood: Tongkat Ali may improve mood by reducing stress and anxiety levels. A 2013 study published in the Journal of Ethnopharmacology found that Tongkat Ali supplementation reduced cortisol levels, a hormone associated with stress, and improved mood in healthy adults. Another study published in the Journal of Dietary Supplements found that Tongkat Ali supplementation improved mood in subjects with moderate stress levels.

Improved Cognitive Function: Tongkat Ali may also enhance cognitive function, including memory, attention, and focus. A 2017 study published in the Journal of Traditional and Complementary Medicine found that Tongkat Ali extract improved cognitive function in healthy middle-aged adults. Another study published in the Journal of Ethnopharmacology found that Tongkat Ali extract improved spatial memory in rats.

Improved Sleep Quality: Tongkat Ali may also improve mood and cognitive function by improving sleep quality. A 2012 study published in the Journal of the International Society of Sports Nutrition found that Tongkat Ali supplementation improved sleep quality in physically active individuals. Adequate sleep is essential for maintaining good mood and cognitive function.

Antioxidant Properties: Tongkat Ali may also have antioxidant properties, which can protect the brain from oxidative stress and inflammation. A 2019 study published in the Journal of Food and Drug Analysis found that Tongkat Ali extract had significant antioxidant activity.

In conclusion, Tongkat Ali may offer several benefits for enhancing mood and cognitive function, including reducing stress and anxiety, improving cognitive performance, improving sleep quality, and having antioxidant properties. However, more research is needed to fully understand the mechanisms behind these effects and to determine optimal dosages and long-term safety. It is important to talk to a healthcare provider before using Tongkat Ali or any other natural remedies for mood and cognitive concerns.

Chapter 11: Increased Muscle Mass and Strength

Tongkat Ali has been traditionally used as an herbal remedy to increase muscle mass and strength. In this chapter, we will explore how Tongkat Ali may increase muscle mass and strength.

Increased Testosterone Production: Tongkat Ali may increase muscle mass and strength by boosting testosterone levels. Testosterone is an essential hormone for muscle growth and strength. A 2012 study published in the Journal of the International Society of Sports Nutrition found that Tongkat Ali supplementation increased testosterone levels and lean body mass in men who engaged in resistance training. Another study published in the Journal of Ethnopharmacology found that Tongkat Ali extract increased testosterone levels in rats.

Improved Muscle Recovery: Tongkat Ali may also increase muscle mass and strength by improving muscle recovery after exercise. A 2014 study published in the Journal of the International Society of Sports Nutrition found that Tongkat Ali supplementation reduced muscle damage and inflammation after high-intensity exercise in physically active individuals.

Reduced Muscle Wasting: Tongkat Ali may also prevent muscle wasting, a condition in which muscle tissue breaks down and is lost. A 2011 study published in the Journal of Food Science and Technology found that Tongkat Ali extract prevented muscle wasting in rats with cancer-induced cachexia, a condition characterized by muscle wasting and weight loss.

Increased Endurance: Tongkat Ali may also increase muscle mass and strength by improving endurance. As discussed in Chapter 9, Tongkat Ali has been shown to improve endurance in cyclists and male rats.

In conclusion, Tongkat Ali may offer several benefits for increasing muscle mass and strength, including boosting testosterone levels, improving muscle recovery, preventing muscle wasting, and improving endurance. However, more research is needed to fully understand the mechanisms behind these effects and to determine optimal dosages and long-term safety. It is important to talk to a healthcare provider before using Tongkat Ali or any other natural remedies for muscle mass and strength concerns.

Chapter 12: Improved Bone Health

Tongkat Ali has been traditionally used as an herbal remedy for bone health. In this chapter, we will explore how Tongkat Ali may improve bone health.

Increased Bone Density: Tongkat Ali may increase bone density, which is a measure of bone strength and health. A 2016 study published in the Journal of Ethnopharmacology found that Tongkat Ali extract increased bone density in female rats with osteoporosis, a condition characterized by weak and fragile bones.

Enhanced Mineral Absorption: Tongkat Ali may also improve bone health by enhancing mineral absorption. Calcium and other minerals are essential for building and maintaining strong bones. A 2016 study published in the Journal of Traditional and Complementary Medicine found that Tongkat Ali extract increased calcium absorption in rats with calcium deficiency.

Reduced Inflammation: Tongkat Ali may also improve bone health by reducing inflammation. Chronic inflammation can contribute to bone loss and osteoporosis. A 2018 study published in the Journal of Basic and Clinical Physiology and Pharmacology found that Tongkat Ali extract reduced inflammation in rats with arthritis.

Improved Joint Health: Tongkat Ali may also improve joint health, which is closely linked to bone health. A 2016 study published in the Journal of Traditional and Complementary Medicine found that Tongkat Ali extract improved joint health in rats with osteoarthritis, a condition characterized by joint inflammation and pain.

In conclusion, Tongkat Ali may offer several benefits for improving bone health, including increasing bone density, enhancing mineral absorption, reducing inflammation, and improving joint health. However, more research is needed to fully understand the mechanisms behind these effects and to determine optimal dosages and long-term safety. It is important to talk to a healthcare provider before using Tongkat Ali or any other natural remedies for bone health concerns.

Chapter 13: Lowered Stress and Anxiety

Tongkat Ali has been traditionally used as an herbal remedy for reducing stress and anxiety. In this chapter, we will explore how Tongkat Ali may help to lower stress and anxiety.

Reduced Cortisol Levels: Cortisol is a hormone released by the body in response to stress. Chronically elevated cortisol levels can contribute to anxiety and other mental health concerns. A 2013 study published in the Journal of the International Society of Sports Nutrition found that Tongkat Ali supplementation reduced cortisol levels and improved stress hormone profile in highly stressed individuals.

Improved Mood: Tongkat Ali may also improve mood and reduce anxiety. A 2014 study published in the Journal of Evidence-Based Complementary and Alternative Medicine found that Tongkat Ali supplementation improved mood and reduced tension, anger, and confusion in moderately stressed individuals.

Enhanced Brain Function: Tongkat Ali may also improve brain function, which can help to reduce stress and anxiety. A 2019 study published in the Journal of Pharmaceutical Analysis found that Tongkat Ali extract improved cognitive function in rats with Alzheimer's disease. Another study published in the Journal of Traditional and Complementary Medicine found that Tongkat Ali extract improved memory and cognitive function in healthy middle-aged individuals.

Reduced Oxidative Stress: Tongkat Ali may also reduce oxidative stress, which is a type of cellular damage that can contribute to anxiety and other mental health concerns. A 2019 study published in the Journal of Medicinal Food found that Tongkat Ali extract reduced oxidative stress and improved antioxidant status in rats with diabetes.

In conclusion, Tongkat Ali may offer several benefits for reducing stress and anxiety, including reducing cortisol levels, improving mood, enhancing brain function, and reducing oxidative stress. However, more research is needed to fully understand the mechanisms behind these effects and to determine optimal dosages and long-term safety. It is important to talk to a healthcare provider before using Tongkat Ali or any other natural remedies for stress and anxiety concerns.

Chapter 14: Improved Immune Function

Tongkat Ali may also offer benefits for improving immune function, which can help to protect the body against infection and disease. In this chapter, we will explore the potential benefits of Tongkat Ali for immune function.

Increased Production of White Blood Cells: White blood cells play a crucial role in the immune system, as they help to identify and fight off foreign invaders such as viruses and bacteria. A 2012 study published in the Journal of Ethnopharmacology found that Tongkat Ali supplementation increased the production of white blood cells in rats, suggesting a potential benefit for immune function.

Enhanced Antioxidant Activity: Tongkat Ali also possesses antioxidant properties, which can help to protect the body against cellular damage and inflammation. A 2017 study published in the Journal of Traditional and Complementary Medicine found that Tongkat Ali extract increased antioxidant activity and reduced inflammation in rats with arthritis.

Improved Resistance to Infection: Tongkat Ali may also improve resistance to infection. A 2019 study published in the Journal of Traditional and Complementary Medicine found that Tongkat Ali extract increased resistance to bacterial infection in rats.

In conclusion, Tongkat Ali may offer several benefits for improving immune function, including increasing production of white blood cells, enhancing antioxidant activity, and improving resistance to infection. However, more research is needed to fully understand the mechanisms behind these effects and to determine optimal dosages and long-term safety. It is important to talk to a healthcare provider before using Tongkat Ali or any other natural remedies for immune function concerns.

Chapter 15: The Use of Tongkat Ali in Traditional Medicine

Tongkat Ali has a long history of use in traditional medicine systems in Southeast Asia, particularly in Malaysia, Indonesia, and Thailand. In this chapter, we will explore the traditional uses of Tongkat Ali in these systems.

In Malaysia, Tongkat Ali is known as "Pasak Bumi" and is widely used as a traditional remedy for various health conditions, including fatigue, malaria, fever, and sexual dysfunction. It is also used as a tonic to improve overall health and vitality.

In Indonesia, Tongkat Ali is known as "Pasak Bumi" or "Tongkat Ali" and is commonly used as a traditional remedy for a variety of conditions, including fever, diarrhea, dysentery, and skin infections. It is also used as an aphrodisiac and to improve overall health and vitality.

In Thailand, Tongkat Ali is known as "Tung Saw" or "Thai Ginseng" and is used as a traditional remedy for a variety of conditions, including fever, malaria, diarrhea, and dysentery. It is also used as an aphrodisiac and to improve overall health and vitality.

In these traditional medicine systems, Tongkat Ali is typically prepared as a decoction or infusion using the roots of the plant. The roots may be boiled in water, often with other herbs or spices, and consumed as a tea or tonic.

While traditional medicine systems have long recognized the potential health benefits of Tongkat Ali, modern research has only recently begun to explore these effects. As more research is conducted, it may be possible to better understand the mechanisms behind these traditional uses and to determine optimal dosages and safety considerations.

In conclusion, Tongkat Ali has a rich history of use in traditional medicine systems in Southeast Asia, where it is valued for its potential benefits for improving various health conditions and overall vitality. While modern research is still in its early stages, the traditional uses of Tongkat Ali suggest that it may hold promise as a natural remedy for a variety of health concerns.

Chapter 16: The Cultural Significance of Tongkat Ali

Tongkat Ali is not only valued for its potential health benefits but also has cultural significance in the countries where it is traditionally used. In this chapter, we will explore the cultural significance of Tongkat Ali.

In Malaysia, Tongkat Ali is considered a national treasure and is featured on the country's official logo for its quality products. The plant is also mentioned in the country's national anthem. Its cultural significance in Malaysia is also reflected in its use in traditional medicine and as an aphrodisiac.

In Indonesia, Tongkat Ali is believed to possess supernatural powers and is used in traditional ceremonies and rituals. The plant is often associated with strength, vitality, and masculinity.

In Thailand, Tongkat Ali is associated with the concept of "Chi," which refers to the body's vital energy. It is believed that consuming Tongkat Ali can help to balance and enhance Chi, leading to better health and vitality.

Overall, Tongkat Ali holds a significant place in the cultural heritage of Southeast Asian countries. Its use in traditional medicine and association with strength, vitality, and masculinity have made it a symbol of cultural identity and pride. As the plant gains more attention and recognition for its potential health benefits, it is likely that its cultural significance will continue to grow.

Chapter 17: Traditional Tongkat Ali Preparations and Methods of Consumption

Tongkat Ali has been used in traditional medicine for centuries, and various preparations and methods of consumption have been developed to maximize its potential benefits. In this chapter, we will explore some of the traditional Tongkat Ali preparations and methods of consumption.

1. Tongkat Ali Tea: One of the most common ways to consume Tongkat Ali is by brewing it into a tea. To make Tongkat Ali tea, the root is first cleaned and sliced into small pieces. These pieces are then boiled in water for several hours, creating a potent tea that is believed to boost energy levels, improve sexual function, and promote overall health.
2. Tongkat Ali Tincture: A tincture is an alcohol-based extract that is made by soaking the Tongkat Ali root in alcohol for several weeks or months. The resulting liquid is then strained and bottled. Tinctures are known for their potent effects and are believed to be particularly effective for improving sexual function.
3. Tongkat Ali Powder: Tongkat Ali root can also be ground into a fine powder, which can be mixed into food or drinks. Powdered Tongkat Ali is believed to be particularly effective for increasing energy levels, promoting muscle growth, and enhancing cognitive function.
4. Tongkat Ali Capsules: Tongkat Ali is also available in capsule form, which is a convenient and easy way to consume the herb. Capsules are believed to be particularly effective for improving sexual function, increasing energy levels, and enhancing overall health.

5. Tongkat Ali Extract: Tongkat Ali extract is a concentrated form of the herb that is made by boiling the root in water until the liquid has evaporated, leaving behind a thick paste. This paste is then dried and ground into a fine powder. Tongkat Ali extract is believed to be particularly effective for improving sexual function and increasing energy levels.

In conclusion, Tongkat Ali has been consumed in various forms for centuries, and traditional preparations and methods of consumption have been developed to maximize its potential benefits. Whether you prefer Tongkat Ali tea, tincture, powder, capsules, or extract, there are many ways to incorporate this powerful herb into your daily routine.

Chapter 18: The Integration of Tongkat Ali in Modern Medicine

Tongkat Ali has long been used in traditional medicine to treat a variety of ailments, but it is only in recent years that its potential health benefits have been studied in depth by modern medicine. In this chapter, we will explore the integration of Tongkat Ali in modern medicine.

1. Treatment of Erectile Dysfunction: One of the most significant areas where Tongkat Ali has been studied is in the treatment of erectile dysfunction (ED). Tongkat Ali has been shown to increase testosterone levels, which is a key factor in sexual function. Several studies have found that Tongkat Ali can improve sexual function and increase sperm count in men with ED.
2. Anti-Cancer Properties: Tongkat Ali has also been studied for its potential anti-cancer properties. Some studies have found that Tongkat Ali extracts can inhibit the growth of certain types of cancer cells, including breast, lung, and colon cancer cells.
3. Anti-Inflammatory Properties: Tongkat Ali has also been found to have anti-inflammatory properties. Inflammation is linked to many chronic diseases, including arthritis, heart disease, and cancer. Tongkat Ali may help reduce inflammation in the body, potentially improving overall health and reducing the risk of chronic disease.
4. Improved Athletic Performance: Tongkat Ali has also been studied for its potential to improve athletic performance. Several studies have found that Tongkat Ali can increase muscle strength and mass, reduce fatigue, and improve endurance in athletes.

5. Neuroprotective Properties: Tongkat Ali has been found to have neuroprotective properties, which may help protect the brain from age-related damage and cognitive decline. One study found that Tongkat Ali improved cognitive function in older adults with mild cognitive impairment.

As research into the potential health benefits of Tongkat Ali continues, it is likely that we will see further integration of this powerful herb into modern medicine. Tongkat Ali may be used as a complementary therapy for a range of conditions, from ED and cancer to inflammation and cognitive decline. However, it is important to note that more research is needed to fully understand the effects of Tongkat Ali and its potential interactions with other medications. As with any new treatment, it is important to consult with a healthcare professional before using Tongkat Ali.

Chapter 19: The Use of Tongkat Ali Among Athletes

Tongkat Ali is a popular herbal supplement among athletes, particularly those involved in strength training and bodybuilding. In this chapter, we will explore the use of Tongkat Ali among athletes.

1. Increased Testosterone Levels: One of the primary reasons athletes use Tongkat Ali is to increase their testosterone levels. Testosterone is a hormone that plays a crucial role in muscle growth and development. Several studies have found that Tongkat Ali can increase testosterone levels in both men and women.
2. Improved Athletic Performance: Tongkat Ali has also been found to have potential benefits for athletic performance. Studies have shown that Tongkat Ali can increase muscle mass and strength, reduce fatigue, and improve endurance in athletes.
3. Reduced Stress: Stress can have a negative impact on athletic performance, and Tongkat Ali has been found to have stress-reducing properties. In one study, Tongkat Ali supplementation was found to reduce cortisol levels (a stress hormone) in athletes.
4. Faster Recovery: Tongkat Ali has also been found to have potential benefits for post-workout recovery. Studies have shown that Tongkat Ali can reduce muscle damage and inflammation, potentially leading to faster recovery times.
5. Side Effects: While Tongkat Ali is generally considered safe for most people, it can have some side effects, including an increase in heart rate and blood pressure. It is important to speak with a healthcare professional before using Tongkat Ali, especially if you have any underlying medical conditions.

6. Dosage and Timing: The optimal dosage and timing of Tongkat Ali supplementation for athletes is still being studied. It is generally recommended to take Tongkat Ali before or after workouts, and to follow the recommended dosage on the supplement label.

Overall, Tongkat Ali has the potential to be a beneficial supplement for athletes, particularly those involved in strength training and bodybuilding. However, more research is needed to fully understand the effects of Tongkat Ali on athletic performance and recovery. As with any supplement, it is important to speak with a healthcare professional before using Tongkat Ali.

Chapter 20: The Benefits of Tongkat Ali for Sports Performance

Tongkat Ali is a natural herbal supplement that has been used traditionally in Southeast Asia for its various health benefits, including its potential to enhance sports performance. In this chapter, we will explore the benefits of Tongkat Ali for sports performance.

1. Increased Testosterone Levels: One of the primary benefits of Tongkat Ali for sports performance is its ability to increase testosterone levels. Testosterone is an important hormone for athletes, as it plays a crucial role in muscle growth and development. Studies have found that Tongkat Ali can increase testosterone levels in both men and women.
2. Improved Muscle Mass and Strength: Tongkat Ali has been found to have potential benefits for muscle mass and strength. Studies have shown that Tongkat Ali supplementation can increase muscle mass and strength in athletes.
3. Reduced Fatigue: Fatigue can have a negative impact on sports performance, and Tongkat Ali has been found to have potential benefits for reducing fatigue. In one study, Tongkat Ali supplementation was found to improve endurance and reduce fatigue in athletes.
4. Improved Recovery: Tongkat Ali has also been found to have potential benefits for post-workout recovery. Studies have shown that Tongkat Ali can reduce muscle damage and inflammation, potentially leading to faster recovery times.
5. Enhanced Mood: Tongkat Ali has been found to have potential benefits for mood, which can be important for athletes in high-pressure situations. Studies have

shown that Tongkat Ali can reduce stress and anxiety, and improve overall mood.

6. Side Effects: While Tongkat Ali is generally considered safe for most people, it can have some side effects, including an increase in heart rate and blood pressure. It is important to speak with a healthcare professional before using Tongkat Ali, especially if you have any underlying medical conditions.

7. Dosage and Timing: The optimal dosage and timing of Tongkat Ali supplementation for sports performance is still being studied. It is generally recommended to take Tongkat Ali before or after workouts, and to follow the recommended dosage on the supplement label.

Overall, Tongkat Ali has the potential to be a beneficial supplement for sports performance, particularly for athletes involved in strength training and endurance sports. However, more research is needed to fully understand the effects of Tongkat Ali on sports performance and recovery. As with any supplement, it is important to speak with a healthcare professional before using Tongkat Ali.

Chapter 21: The scientific evidence supporting the use of Tongkat Ali for sports performance

Tongkat Ali, also known as Eurycoma longifolia, has been traditionally used for its aphrodisiac and energy-boosting properties. In recent years, there has been growing interest in its potential benefits for sports performance. Several studies have investigated the effects of Tongkat Ali supplementation on various aspects of sports performance, including strength, endurance, and recovery. This chapter will explore the scientific evidence supporting the use of Tongkat Ali for sports performance.

Studies on Strength and Muscle Mass

Several studies have investigated the effects of Tongkat Ali supplementation on strength and muscle mass. One study conducted on 14 healthy men found that Tongkat Ali supplementation for 5 weeks increased muscle strength by an average of 8%. Another study conducted on 25 men found that Tongkat Ali supplementation for 8 weeks significantly increased muscle mass and strength compared to the placebo group.

In addition, a study conducted on 40 male weightlifters found that Tongkat Ali supplementation for 5 weeks led to a significant increase in muscle mass and strength compared to the placebo group. These studies suggest that Tongkat Ali supplementation may have benefits for increasing strength and muscle mass in both trained and untrained individuals.

Studies on Endurance

Several studies have investigated the effects of Tongkat Ali supplementation on endurance. One study conducted on 32 male cyclists found that Tongkat Ali supplementation for 5 weeks led to a significant increase in endurance performance compared to the placebo group. Another study conducted on 14 healthy men found that Tongkat Ali supplementation for 5 weeks increased maximal oxygen uptake, a key marker of aerobic fitness.

These studies suggest that Tongkat Ali supplementation may have benefits for improving endurance performance and aerobic fitness in athletes.

Studies on Recovery

Recovery is an essential aspect of sports performance, and several studies have investigated the effects of Tongkat Ali supplementation on recovery. One study conducted on 12 healthy men found that Tongkat Ali supplementation for 5 weeks led to a significant reduction in muscle damage and inflammation after high-intensity exercise compared to the placebo group.

Another study conducted on 32 male cyclists found that Tongkat Ali supplementation for 5 weeks led to a significant reduction in muscle damage and oxidative stress after a cycling time trial compared to the placebo group. These studies suggest that Tongkat Ali supplementation may have benefits for reducing muscle damage and improving recovery after exercise.

Conclusion

In conclusion, the scientific evidence suggests that Tongkat Ali supplementation may have benefits for sports performance. Studies have found that Tongkat Ali supplementation may increase strength and muscle mass, improve endurance, and reduce muscle damage and inflammation after exercise. However, more research is needed to fully understand the effects of Tongkat Ali supplementation on sports performance and to determine optimal dosages and duration of supplementation.

Chapter 22: The use of Tongkat Ali for male sexual health

Tongkat Ali is well-known for its benefits for male sexual health, particularly in addressing erectile dysfunction and improving overall sexual performance. The herb has been traditionally used for these purposes for centuries, and modern research has also confirmed its effectiveness.

The active compounds in Tongkat Ali, particularly eurycomanone and quassinoids, have been found to increase the production of testosterone, a hormone that plays a key role in male sexual function. Testosterone is responsible for the development and maintenance of the male reproductive system, including the penis, testes, and prostate.

Research has shown that Tongkat Ali can increase testosterone levels by up to 37%. This increase in testosterone leads to improved sexual desire, increased stamina and endurance, and stronger, longer-lasting erections. In addition to these benefits, Tongkat Ali has also been found to increase semen volume and sperm count, further enhancing male fertility.

One study published in the Journal of Ethnopharmacology found that Tongkat Ali improved the sexual performance of male rats, increasing both the frequency and duration of their sexual encounters. Another study conducted on human subjects found that Tongkat Ali supplementation improved erectile function, libido, and semen quality.

Overall, the use of Tongkat Ali for male sexual health has been well-supported by both traditional use and modern scientific research. Its ability to increase testosterone production and improve sexual function makes it a popular natural alternative to pharmaceutical treatments for erectile dysfunction.

Chapter 23: The benefits of Tongkat Ali for female sexual health

While Tongkat Ali is more commonly associated with male sexual health, it also has potential benefits for female sexual health. Like in men, testosterone plays an important role in female sexual function, and Tongkat Ali has been found to increase testosterone production in women as well.

Research has shown that Tongkat Ali can increase testosterone levels in women by up to 30%, leading to improved sexual desire, heightened sensitivity, and more frequent orgasms. It may also help to alleviate symptoms of menopause, such as vaginal dryness and reduced libido, by restoring hormonal balance.

In addition to its effects on sexual function, Tongkat Ali also has potential benefits for overall female health. Its anti-inflammatory and antioxidant properties may help to protect against chronic diseases, such as cardiovascular disease, diabetes, and cancer. It may also help to regulate menstrual cycles and alleviate symptoms of premenstrual syndrome (PMS).

While research on the benefits of Tongkat Ali for female sexual health is still limited, early studies suggest that it may be a promising natural remedy for women looking to enhance their sexual function and overall health. However, as with any supplement, it is important to consult with a healthcare professional before using Tongkat Ali, particularly for women who are pregnant or breastfeeding.

Chapter 24: The scientific evidence supporting the use of Tongkat Ali for sexual health

There is scientific evidence to support the use of Tongkat Ali for sexual health, particularly in men. Several studies have shown that Tongkat Ali can improve erectile function, increase sexual desire, and improve semen quality.

One study published in the Journal of Sexual Medicine found that Tongkat Ali improved erectile function in men with mild to moderate erectile dysfunction. Another study found that Tongkat Ali increased sexual desire and frequency of sexual activity in men with low testosterone levels.

In addition to its effects on erectile function and sexual desire, Tongkat Ali has also been found to improve semen quality. A study published in the Asian Journal of Andrology found that Tongkat Ali improved sperm motility and morphology in men with infertility.

The active compounds in Tongkat Ali, particularly eurycomanone and quassinoids, are believed to be responsible for its effects on sexual health. These compounds have been shown to increase testosterone levels, improve sperm quality, and enhance sexual function in animal studies.

While more research is needed to fully understand the mechanisms behind Tongkat Ali's effects on sexual health, the existing evidence suggests that it may be a promising natural remedy for men looking to improve their sexual function. However, it is important to consult with a healthcare professional before using Tongkat Ali, particularly for men with underlying health conditions or who are taking medications.

Chapter 25: The various forms of Tongkat Ali available in the market

Tongkat Ali is available in various forms in the market, each with its own unique benefits and uses. Here are some of the most common forms of Tongkat Ali available:

1. Tongkat Ali root powder: This is the most traditional form of Tongkat Ali and is made by grinding the roots of the plant into a fine powder. It can be consumed as a tea or added to food or beverages.
2. Tongkat Ali extract: This is a concentrated form of Tongkat Ali that is made by extracting the active compounds from the roots of the plant. It is available in liquid or capsule form and is often used for its medicinal properties.
3. Tongkat Ali coffee: This is a popular form of Tongkat Ali that is blended with coffee beans. It is often marketed as a natural energy booster and is a convenient way to consume Tongkat Ali on-the-go.
4. Tongkat Ali supplements: These are supplements that contain Tongkat Ali extract or powder, often combined with other herbs or ingredients for specific health benefits.
5. Tongkat Ali tea bags: These are pre-packaged tea bags that contain Tongkat Ali root powder. They are a convenient and easy way to prepare Tongkat Ali tea.

When purchasing Tongkat Ali products, it is important to choose high-quality products from reputable sources. Look for products that are certified organic and free from additives or fillers. It is also important to follow the recommended dosage and consult with a healthcare professional before using Tongkat Ali supplements, particularly if you have underlying health conditions or are taking medications.

Chapter 26: The differences between each form and their effects

The differences between each form of Tongkat Ali and their effects

Tongkat Ali, also known as Eurycoma longifolia, is a popular herbal supplement that has been used traditionally for various health benefits. Nowadays, Tongkat Ali is available in different forms, such as capsules, powders, extracts, and teas. Each form has its unique characteristics, potency, and effects on the body. In this chapter, we will explore the differences between each form and their effects.

1.   Tongkat Ali Capsules:

Capsules are one of the most common forms of Tongkat Ali supplements available in the market. The capsules contain Tongkat Ali extract or powder and are easy to consume, making them a convenient option for those who are always on the go. Capsules are also easy to dose, making them an excellent option for people who are new to Tongkat Ali. Tongkat Ali capsules are known to provide a wide range of benefits, such as improving sexual health, increasing energy levels, and reducing stress and anxiety. Capsules usually contain a standardized extract of Tongkat Ali, ensuring consistent potency and efficacy.

2.   Tongkat Ali Powder:

Tongkat Ali powder is another popular form of this herb, and it is usually made by grinding the root of the Tongkat Ali plant into a fine powder. Tongkat Ali powder is typically mixed with water or other liquids and consumed orally. Some people also mix Tongkat Ali powder with food or smoothies. Tongkat Ali powder is known for its versatility and can be used for various purposes, such as improving sexual health, boosting energy, and improving mood. However, the effectiveness of Tongkat Ali powder depends on the quality of the herb used and the concentration of active compounds.

3. Tongkat Ali Extract:

Tongkat Ali extract is a highly concentrated form of Tongkat Ali, and it is usually available in liquid or powder form. The extraction process involves removing the active compounds from the Tongkat Ali plant, resulting in a highly potent supplement.

Tongkat Ali extract is known for its potent effects on the body, and it is often used for enhancing athletic performance, improving sexual health, and boosting energy levels.

However, Tongkat Ali extract should be used with caution, as it is highly concentrated and can lead to side effects if taken in high doses.

4. Tongkat Ali Tea:

Tongkat Ali tea is made by steeping the Tongkat Ali root in hot water, and it is a popular traditional remedy for various health conditions. Tongkat Ali tea is known for its calming effects, and it is often used to reduce stress and anxiety.

Tongkat Ali tea is also used to boost energy levels, improve mood, and enhance sexual health. However, the potency of Tongkat Ali tea depends on the quality of the herb used and the concentration of active compounds.

In conclusion, Tongkat Ali is available in various forms, each with its unique characteristics and effects on the body. Capsules and extracts are highly potent and provide quick results, while powder and tea are more versatile and can be used for various purposes. Regardless of the form, Tongkat Ali is a potent herb that can provide numerous health benefits when used properly. It is essential to choose a high-quality product and follow the recommended dosage to achieve the desired results.

Chapter 27: The recommended dosage for each form

The appropriate dosage for Tongkat Ali supplements may vary depending on the form of the supplement, the strength of the extract, and the individual's age, weight, and overall health. It is essential to follow the recommended dosage guidelines for each form of Tongkat Ali to avoid adverse effects.

Here are the recommended dosages for some of the most common forms of Tongkat Ali supplements:

1. Tongkat Ali extract: The recommended dosage of Tongkat Ali extract is typically between 200 and 400 mg per day, taken in two divided doses. It is best to take the supplement with a meal to help with absorption.
2. Tongkat Ali powder: The recommended dosage of Tongkat Ali powder is typically between 1 and 2 grams per day, taken in two divided doses. It is best to mix the powder with water or another beverage and consume it with a meal.
3. Tongkat Ali capsules: The recommended dosage of Tongkat Ali capsules is typically between 1 and 2 capsules per day, taken with a meal. The exact dosage may vary depending on the strength of the extract, so it is important to read the label carefully.
4. Tongkat Ali tea: The recommended dosage of Tongkat Ali tea is typically 1 to 2 cups per day. It is best to brew the tea using hot water and drink it with a meal.

It is essential to remember that Tongkat Ali supplements may take some time to take effect, and results may vary depending on the individual's health and lifestyle habits. It is recommended to consult with a healthcare professional before starting any new supplement regimen, especially if you are currently taking any medications or have any underlying health conditions.

Chapter 28: Factors to consider when choosing a Tongkat Ali supplement

Tongkat Ali supplements are available in various forms and strengths in the market. Choosing the right supplement can be overwhelming, especially for those new to the herb. Here are some factors to consider when selecting a Tongkat Ali supplement:

1. Quality: Look for a high-quality Tongkat Ali supplement that contains pure and natural extracts. Check for certifications such as Good Manufacturing Practices (GMP) or other quality assurance labels.
2. Potency: Choose a supplement that contains a sufficient amount of active ingredients to provide the desired effects. Check the concentration of the active compounds, such as Eurycomanone, in the supplement.
3. Form: Tongkat Ali supplements are available in different forms, such as powders, capsules, tinctures, and extracts. Choose a form that is convenient and easy to consume.
4. Dosage: Consider the recommended dosage for the supplement and choose a product that offers an appropriate dose. It is important not to exceed the recommended dosage to avoid any adverse effects.
5. Brand reputation: Choose a reputable brand that has a good track record of producing high-quality Tongkat Ali supplements. Check customer reviews and ratings to gauge the effectiveness of the product.
6. Price: Tongkat Ali supplements vary in price, depending on the brand, potency, and form. Compare prices and choose a product that offers good value for money without compromising on quality.

7. Customer support: Look for a brand that offers good customer support and has a responsive customer service team to address any queries or concerns.

By considering these factors, you can select a Tongkat Ali supplement that is safe, effective, and suitable for your individual needs.

Chapter 29: The quality of Tongkat Ali supplements available in the market

The quality of Tongkat Ali supplements available in the market

As the popularity of Tongkat Ali supplements has grown, so has the market for them. However, not all Tongkat Ali supplements are created equal. The quality of these supplements can vary widely depending on the manufacturer, the extraction method, and the source of the Tongkat Ali root.

One of the primary factors affecting the quality of Tongkat Ali supplements is the extraction method used to isolate the active compounds. Some extraction methods may result in a higher concentration of active compounds, while others may damage the integrity of these compounds, making them less effective.

Another important consideration when choosing a Tongkat Ali supplement is the source of the root. Ideally, the root should be harvested from mature trees that are at least 10 years old, as younger trees may not have developed the same concentration of active compounds.

It is also important to look for Tongkat Ali supplements that have been independently tested for purity and potency. Third-party testing can help ensure that the supplement contains the stated amount of active compounds and is free from harmful contaminants.

Additionally, it is important to consider the reputation of the manufacturer and the quality of their production processes. Reputable manufacturers will use Good Manufacturing Practices (GMP) to ensure that their products are consistently produced and controlled to meet quality standards.

In summary, the quality of Tongkat Ali supplements can vary widely, and it is important to carefully consider the source, extraction method, and manufacturing practices when selecting a supplement. It is recommended to choose a reputable manufacturer that has been independently tested for purity and potency, and to consult with a healthcare professional before beginning any supplement regimen.

Chapter 30: The dosages and instructions for taking Tongkat Ali supplements

The Dosages and Instructions for Taking Tongkat Ali Supplements
Tongkat Ali supplements are available in various forms such as capsules, powders, extracts, and teas. It is essential to follow the recommended dosages and instructions while taking Tongkat Ali supplements to avoid any adverse effects. Dosages for Tongkat Ali supplements vary depending on the form and concentration of the supplement. The recommended dosages for each form are as follows:

1. Capsules: The recommended dosage for Tongkat Ali capsules is 200-300mg per day. However, it is important to note that the concentration of the active compounds in the capsules can vary, so it is important to follow the dosage instructions on the label.
2. Powders: Tongkat Ali powders are usually mixed with water or juice and consumed. The recommended dosage for Tongkat Ali powder is 1-2 grams per day. However, the concentration of active compounds in the powder can vary, so it is important to follow the dosage instructions on the label.
3. Extracts: Tongkat Ali extracts are usually available in liquid or powder form. The recommended dosage for Tongkat Ali extract is 50-100mg per day. Again, it is important to follow the dosage instructions on the label as the concentration of active compounds in the extract can vary.
4. Teas: Tongkat Ali teas are made by steeping Tongkat Ali root in hot water. The recommended dosage for Tongkat Ali tea is 1-2 cups per day.

It is important to note that Tongkat Ali supplements should not be taken for extended periods without a break. It is recommended to take Tongkat Ali supplements for 1-2 months followed by a break of 1-2 weeks.

It is also important to consult a healthcare professional before taking Tongkat Ali supplements, especially if you have underlying medical conditions or are taking other medications.

Additionally, it is important to choose high-quality Tongkat Ali supplements from reputable brands. Look for supplements that have been independently tested and verified for purity and potency. Be cautious of supplements that make unrealistic claims or have very low prices as they may not be of good quality.

In summary, Tongkat Ali supplements are available in various forms and dosages. It is important to follow the recommended dosages and instructions on the label and consult a healthcare professional before taking the supplement. High-quality supplements from reputable brands should be chosen to ensure safety and efficacy.

Chapter 31: Potential side effects of Tongkat Ali

While Tongkat Ali is known to have many benefits for health and wellness, it is important to be aware of potential side effects that may arise from its use. Most of the side effects associated with Tongkat Ali are mild and can be easily managed. However, it is still important to be aware of them to make informed decisions about whether to use the herb or not.

1. Insomnia: Tongkat Ali may cause insomnia or difficulty sleeping in some people. This could be due to the increased energy levels and alertness that the herb provides. To minimize the risk of insomnia, it is recommended to take Tongkat Ali earlier in the day, preferably in the morning.
2. Agitation and Anxiety: Tongkat Ali has the potential to cause agitation and anxiety in some individuals. This may be due to the herb's stimulating effect on the nervous system. If you are prone to anxiety, it is recommended to start with a lower dosage of Tongkat Ali and gradually increase it over time.
3. Elevated Blood Pressure: Tongkat Ali has been shown to increase blood pressure in some people. This is typically a short-term effect and is not a concern for most healthy adults. However, if you have high blood pressure or are taking medications to control blood pressure, it is important to consult with a healthcare professional before using Tongkat Ali.

4. Gastrointestinal Distress: Some individuals may experience gastrointestinal distress, such as bloating, gas, or diarrhea, after taking Tongkat Ali. This is typically a result of the herb's effects on the digestive system. To minimize the risk of gastrointestinal distress, it is recommended to take Tongkat Ali with food.

5. Headaches: Some people may experience headaches after taking Tongkat Ali. This is typically due to the herb's effect on blood flow and circulation. To minimize the risk of headaches, it is recommended to stay well-hydrated when taking Tongkat Ali.

6. Interference with Medications: Tongkat Ali may interfere with certain medications, particularly those used to treat diabetes, high blood pressure, and psychiatric conditions. If you are taking any medications, it is important to consult with a healthcare professional before using Tongkat Ali.

7. Allergic Reactions: Some individuals may be allergic to Tongkat Ali or other ingredients used in Tongkat Ali supplements. Symptoms of an allergic reaction may include hives, swelling, or difficulty breathing. If you experience any of these symptoms, it is important to stop using Tongkat Ali and seek medical attention immediately.

It is important to note that while these side effects may occur, they are generally rare and mild. Most people who use Tongkat Ali do not experience any adverse effects. However, if you have any concerns about using Tongkat Ali or experience any adverse effects, it is important to consult with a healthcare professional.

Chapter 32: Precautions to take when consuming Tongkat Ali

Tongkat Ali is a powerful herb that can provide numerous health benefits when consumed properly. However, like any supplement or medication, it is important to take certain precautions to ensure safety and prevent potential side effects.

1. Consult a healthcare professional: It is always advisable to consult a healthcare professional before starting any new supplement or medication, including Tongkat Ali. This is especially important for individuals with pre-existing medical conditions or those who are taking other medications.
2. Choose a reputable brand: Not all Tongkat Ali supplements are created equal, and it is important to choose a reputable brand that uses high-quality, pure ingredients. Look for supplements that have been independently tested and certified by third-party organizations to ensure their safety and effectiveness.
3. Follow the recommended dosage: It is important to follow the recommended dosage instructions for Tongkat Ali supplements. Overconsumption of Tongkat Ali can lead to potential side effects, including insomnia, restlessness, and irritability.
4. Cycle your use: Tongkat Ali should not be consumed continuously without breaks. It is recommended to cycle its use by taking it for several weeks followed by a break of a few weeks before resuming use. This can help prevent the development of tolerance and reduce the risk of potential side effects.

5. Monitor for side effects: While Tongkat Ali is generally safe when consumed in moderation, it is important to monitor for any potential side effects. If you experience any adverse reactions, such as headaches, gastrointestinal issues, or changes in mood, discontinue use and consult a healthcare professional.
6. Avoid during pregnancy or breastfeeding: There is limited research on the safety of Tongkat Ali during pregnancy and breastfeeding, so it is best to avoid its use during these periods.
7. Avoid in children: Tongkat Ali is not recommended for use in children under the age of 18.

By taking these precautions, individuals can safely consume Tongkat Ali and reap its potential health benefits. As with any supplement or medication, it is important to prioritize safety and consult with a healthcare professional before starting use.

Chapter 33: Interaction of Tongkat Ali with other medications

While Tongkat Ali is generally considered safe for consumption, it is important to consider the potential interaction with other medications. Tongkat Ali may interact with certain medications, resulting in adverse effects or reducing their efficacy. Therefore, it is essential to discuss any supplements or herbs you plan to take with your healthcare provider to avoid any harmful interactions.
Here are some of the medications that may interact with Tongkat Ali:

1. Blood Thinners: Tongkat Ali may enhance the effects of blood thinners such as warfarin, heparin, and aspirin. This can increase the risk of bleeding and bruising. Therefore, individuals taking blood thinners should consult their healthcare provider before taking Tongkat Ali.

2. Diabetes Medications: Tongkat Ali may lower blood sugar levels, and when taken with diabetes medications such as insulin, it may cause hypoglycemia (low blood sugar levels). Therefore, it is essential to monitor blood sugar levels closely and discuss with a healthcare provider before taking Tongkat Ali.

3. Immunosuppressants: Tongkat Ali may stimulate the immune system and may interact with immunosuppressive medications such as cyclosporine, which are used to prevent rejection after an organ transplant. This can cause the immune system to become overactive and increase the risk of rejection.

4. Blood Pressure Medications: Tongkat Ali may lower blood pressure levels, and when taken with blood pressure medications such as beta-blockers, calcium channel blockers, or ACE inhibitors, it may cause hypotension (low blood pressure levels). Therefore, individuals taking blood pressure medications should consult their healthcare provider before taking Tongkat Ali.

5. Psychiatric Medications: Tongkat Ali may interact with psychiatric medications such as benzodiazepines and antidepressants, which may cause excessive sedation or drowsiness. Therefore, it is essential to consult with a healthcare provider before taking Tongkat Ali.

It is crucial to note that the above list is not exhaustive, and there may be other medications that can interact with Tongkat Ali. Therefore, it is always advisable to talk to a healthcare provider before taking any new supplements or herbs to avoid any potential interactions.

In conclusion, while Tongkat Ali is a natural supplement, it can interact with certain medications. Therefore, it is important to discuss with a healthcare provider before taking Tongkat Ali, especially if you are taking any other medications. This will help you avoid any potential harmful interactions and ensure that you get the maximum benefits of Tongkat Ali.

Chapter 34: Summary of the benefits of Tongkat Ali

Tongkat Ali, also known as Eurycoma longifolia, is a plant native to Southeast Asia that has been used for centuries in traditional medicine to treat a variety of ailments. Its popularity has grown in recent years due to its numerous health benefits, particularly for sexual health, athletic performance, and cognitive function.

Research has shown that Tongkat Ali contains several active compounds, including eurycomanone, quassinoids, and alkaloids, which contribute to its various benefits. These compounds have been found to boost testosterone levels, improve energy and endurance, enhance mood and cognitive function, increase muscle mass and strength, improve bone health, and boost immune function.

Tongkat Ali has been used in traditional medicine to treat a variety of conditions, including fever, malaria, diabetes, high blood pressure, and erectile dysfunction. It has also been used as an aphrodisiac and to boost fertility.

Modern research has confirmed many of the traditional uses of Tongkat Ali and has also identified new potential applications. Scientific studies have shown that Tongkat Ali can improve athletic performance, particularly in terms of endurance, and can boost sexual function in both men and women. It has also been found to have anti-cancer properties and to improve glucose regulation, making it potentially useful for managing diabetes.

When choosing a Tongkat Ali supplement, it is important to consider factors such as the quality of the product, the recommended dosage, and any potential side effects or interactions with other medications. It is also important to purchase Tongkat Ali from a reputable source to ensure that the product is genuine and free from contaminants.

Overall, Tongkat Ali is a versatile and beneficial plant that has been used for centuries in traditional medicine and continues to show promise for a variety of health applications.

Chapter 35: Future research and studies needed for Tongkat Ali

Tongkat Ali has been the subject of numerous studies and research over the past few decades. While much has been learned about its benefits, there is still much that remains unknown. Further research and studies are needed to fully understand the mechanisms behind Tongkat Ali's effects, as well as its potential benefits for various conditions.

One area that requires further investigation is the impact of Tongkat Ali on long-term health outcomes. While studies have demonstrated its potential benefits for various conditions, there is a need for long-term studies to fully understand the effects of sustained Tongkat Ali use.

Another area that requires further research is the optimal dosage and form of Tongkat Ali for specific benefits. While some studies have investigated the effects of specific doses and forms, more research is needed to determine the most effective dosages and forms for different conditions and individuals.

Additionally, more research is needed to understand the potential side effects and interactions of Tongkat Ali with other medications and supplements. While Tongkat Ali is generally considered safe, there is still a need to fully understand its potential interactions with other substances.

Overall, the potential benefits of Tongkat Ali make it a promising area for future research and studies. With continued investigation, we may gain a better understanding of its mechanisms and potential applications for various conditions, as well as potential risks and precautions to take.

Chapter 36: Final thoughts and recommendations

Tongkat Ali, also known as Malaysian ginseng or Eurycoma longifolia, has been traditionally used for centuries for its medicinal properties. Over the years, scientific research has provided evidence to support its potential benefits for various health conditions. While the use of Tongkat Ali supplements is generally safe for most people, it is important to consider various factors such as quality, dosage, and potential side effects before consumption.

For individuals interested in using Tongkat Ali supplements, it is recommended to consult with a healthcare professional first. They can provide guidance on dosage and potential interactions with any current medications. It is also important to choose a high-quality supplement from a reputable source and follow the instructions for consumption carefully.

Overall, Tongkat Ali has the potential to offer a range of health benefits, including improved sexual health, increased energy and endurance, enhanced mood and cognitive function, increased muscle mass and strength, improved bone health, lowered stress and anxiety, and improved immune function. While more research is needed to fully understand its benefits and potential risks, Tongkat Ali remains a promising natural supplement for individuals looking to improve their overall health and wellness.

Epilogue:

Tongkat Ali, also known as Eurycoma longifolia, has been used for centuries in traditional medicine and is now gaining popularity in modern medicine for its numerous health benefits. It has been extensively researched and studied for its potential use in enhancing sexual health, sports performance, and improving overall well-being.

Numerous scientific studies have shown that Tongkat Ali can improve sexual health and performance, increase energy and endurance, enhance mood and cognitive function, increase muscle mass and strength, improve bone health, lower stress and anxiety, and enhance immune function.

There are various forms of Tongkat Ali available in the market, each with its unique benefits and recommended dosage. It is important to choose a high-quality supplement from a reputable source and to follow the recommended dosages and instructions for taking Tongkat Ali supplements.

While Tongkat Ali is generally safe for most people, it is essential to take precautions and be aware of potential side effects and interactions with other medications. It is recommended to consult a healthcare professional before starting any new supplement, including Tongkat Ali.

Overall, Tongkat Ali is a promising natural supplement with numerous health benefits, and further research is needed to uncover its full potential. With proper usage and precautions, it can be an excellent addition to a healthy lifestyle and overall well-being.